Furnigore and the Alzheimer's Cure

by

Sid Weiskirch

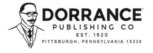
DORRANCE
PUBLISHING CO
EST. 1920
PITTSBURGH, PENNSYLVANIA 15238

Dorrance Publishing Co
585 Alpha Drive
Suite 103
Pittsburgh, PA 15238
Visit our website at *www.dorrancebookstore.com*

ISBN: 978-1-6461-0465-9
eISBN: 978-1-6461-0752-0

THE FURNIGORE PARABLES

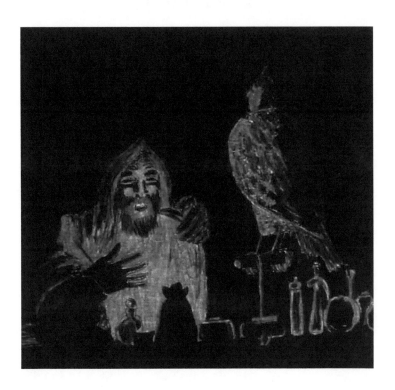

THE ADVENTURES OF FURNIGORE
PART ONE

1. How FURNIGORE can solve the cancer riddle using selective breeding.
2. How FURNIGORE AND ONE ODD PAN help Vladimere Rongnotesksi turn a rock band into a world class symphony orchestra.
3. How FURNIGORE saves the Cleanup Kingdom from disaster.

THE ADVENTURES OF FURNIGORE
PART TWO

1. How FURNIGORE uncovers the biggest presidential campaign scandal of all time.

2. How FURNIGORE stops a worldwide computer hacker attack.

3. How FURNIGORE cures kids from watching too much TV and video games.

4. How FURNIGORE saves One Fat Pan's HI CALORIC restaurant chain.

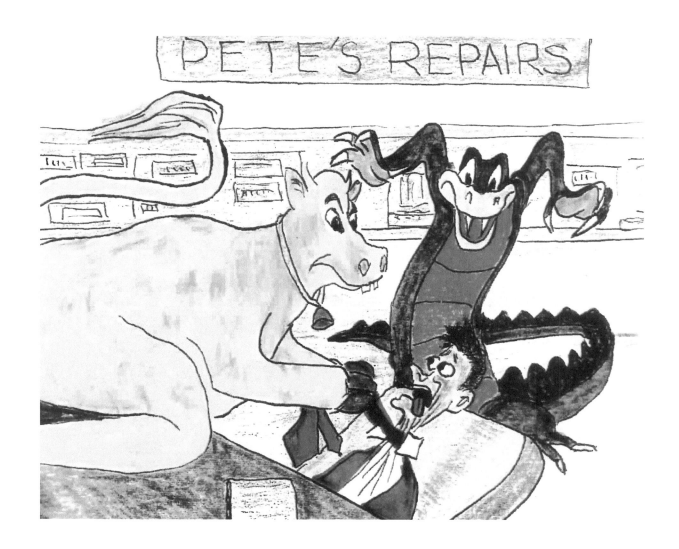

THE ADVENTURES OF FURNIGORE
PART THREE

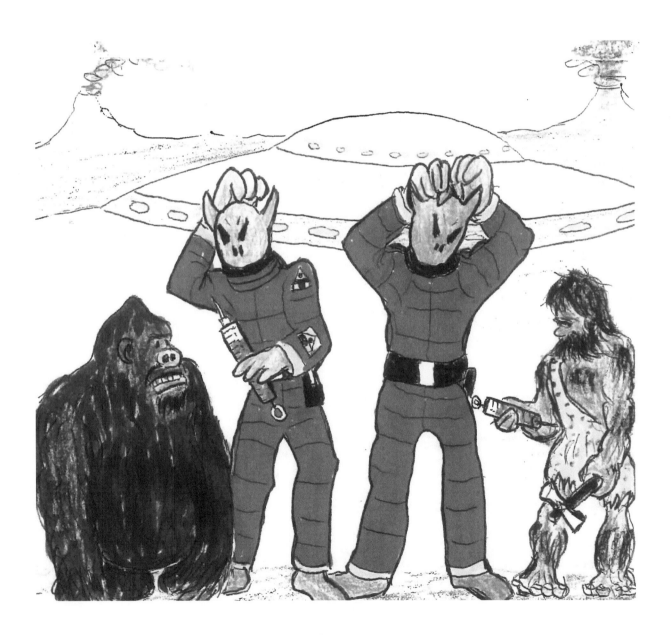

THREE FANTASY STORIES

1. A U.F.O. crashes with thousand-year-old survivors. Is it possible Methusaleh actually lived 900 years?

2. How young TAJIN saves the INCA EMPIRE in Peru.

3. A Reagan era comic collection for today's politicians.

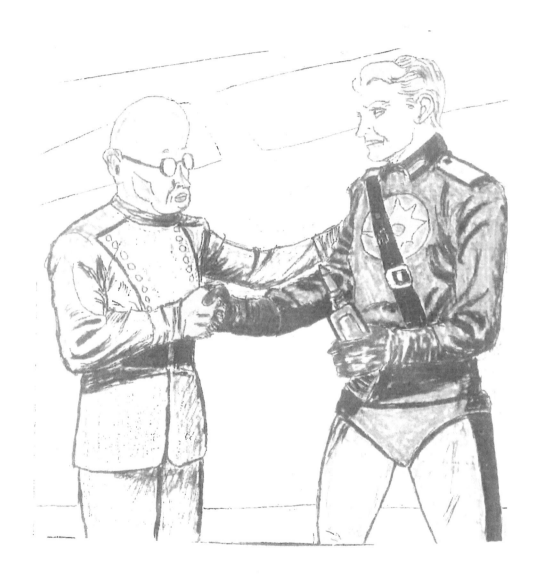

OUT STEPPED THE LIFE FORM THAT WAS RESPONSIBLE FOR PRODUCING THE HUMAN RACE ON OUR PLANET.

PREFACE

Larry is a biology professor in a college in America. Letty, his mother, was a social worker.

Anna, his daughter, is an ER doctor. Ben, his son, is an astronaut with the U.S. Space Agency. Kurt, Larry's father, is a retired businessman. He was Letty's care giver for six years after she contracted Alzheimer's disease. Later, she moved to a nursing home in the Midwest…

Larry's father has been using a one-minute hand warming exercise, called biofeedback, for 60 years to prevent his migraine headaches. He believed that these exercises could help Alzheimer's patients because they flush from the brain the sticky platelets that cause the disease. He hired a helper to coach Letty with the exercises. After only five weeks, the biofeedback exercises were helping her make a recovery…

Unfortunately, she then had a serious fall, and she passed away, ending the exercises just when it appeared there would be an important breakthrough.

Over the past few years, many doctors, psychologists, nurses, and social workers have used these exercises to help many patients with many different illnesses. A huge new industry of professionals, charging $200 an hour developed. (see B.C.I.A) But, no one tried it on Alzheimer's patients.

When Larry's father tried to get the large research foundations to finance a research project to finance a study to prove the value of these exercises, he was blocked for a variety of reasons. It seemed that too many pharmaceutical companies, hospitals, doctors, nursing homes, research foundations, and even biofeedback practitioners, felt it would hurt them financially. If these exercises were successful, anyone could do them…FREE. It was in their best interest to stop or delay the exercises.

PERHAPS LETTY'S FALL WAS NO ACCIDENT?

It was at this point that Larry decided to ask for help from his old friends, One Odd Pan and Furnigore, who lived in the Clean Up Kingdom, in a land far, far, away…in an alternate universe next to our own.

"Welcome back to the Clean Up Kingdom" says Pan.

"Did you come to get away from winter and get a tan?"

Larry says, "It's great to see you all again.

Our winters are all really a pain,

But, it's wonderful, being here, again."

"You all look fine, and I hope things are going well."

Pan says, "You've help us more times than I can tell.

I hope all is well with your mother at home?"

"Unfortunately, the answer is NO," says Larry, with a groan.

"My mother's life ended, when she had a bad fall.

She had Alzheimer's disease, and the fall ended it all.

We were into our fifth week with exercises called biofeedback.

She was getting better, and we hoped she would be back on track.

"These exercises warmed her hands and removed

Problems in her brain.

If we were successful, it could help millions of people

Who are under such terrible strain.

"Unfortunately, many groups, and companies, never

Tried to help us reach our goal.

Many people discouraged us, and even stole.

They felt as long as our exercises were free,

They would lose a lot of money…between you and me."

Pan and Furnigore could not understand how people

Could be so cruel in Larry's land.

Larry says, "Profit is the driving force,

In my land…as a matter course."

Pan says, "I will leave you now for a while.
I'll go to my laboratory, and see what answers I have on file."
Furnigore says, "We will help you solve this problem
Using all our resources."
Larry says, "I'll stay as long as it takes.
Nothing will stop me, not even wild horses."

Pan returns with a victorious smile.
"I used my special powers plus information on file.
I went into a trance and saw the past.
The answers then came quick and fast.
"It seems that there is a large company that
Makes medicines and pills.
Doctors prescribe them and a pharmacist
Fills and refills.

"This company is the culprit in this
Mystery of yours and mine.
Its name is Jones, Sten,
And Von Grumpstein.

"They were about to introduce
A brand-new pill.
It was to cure Parkinson's and Alzheimer's.
You know the drill.

"First, they authorize a 30-
Million-dollar ad campaign,
Then, they plan to make a lot of money
And drink lots of champagne.

"If it became known that Letty's
Trial was a success,
It would bankrupt the company
And cause a mess.

"They decided to delay the five
Week trial at any cost.
If they didn't, the entire company
Would be lost.

"They hired a group of
Ex-professional spies
From an agency that
Deals in crimes and lies.

"They all worked together
To formulate a plan.
If it worked, their company
Would not be an also ran.

"They decided to have one of their agents
Get a job on Letty's nursing home's floor.
She would be her care giver, and help her
Move from floor to floor.

"Her job was to cause Letty to fall
And not hurt her badly.
It was to stop the treatments for a while,
And not end things so sadly.

"Unfortunately, it was not to be that way.
The fall was serious enough to activate
An old heart ailment gone astray,
And poor Letty passed away that very day."
Larry says, "If it can be proven
That the fall was deliberate,
It could be a case of murder.
We must consider it!"

Furnigore says, "How can we
Prove such a thing?"
Pan says, "We must find a way
To make such a charge, really sting."

Larry says, "If we can get Von Grumpstein
To admit his guilt,
We could get him in front of a judge
And watch him wilt."

Pan says, "This would require a plan
Not known in your land.
It would require help from the
Entire Clean Up Clan.

"This will require a visit to Grumpstein
In a dream.
We will terrify him,
And watch him scream.

"After a visit from
Our usual team,
He will be so nervous at the trial,
It will be time to remind him of his dream.
We will make him break down
In front of the judge and jury.
He will be in a state
Of fright and fury."

The scene now shifts to the country club
Where Von Grumpsten plays his golf.
He relaxes with his family
And his dog named Rolf.
After dinner, Arnold Von Grumpstein
Announces that he will take a nap.
He is happy that he stopped the threat to his ads,
And has more promotions on tap.

Von Grumpstein goes to his room
And hears the sounds of distant thunder.
There will be no golf today
To disturb his slumber.

He falls into a blissful sleep,
And hears a knock on his door.
When he opens the door,
He suddenly falls on the floor.

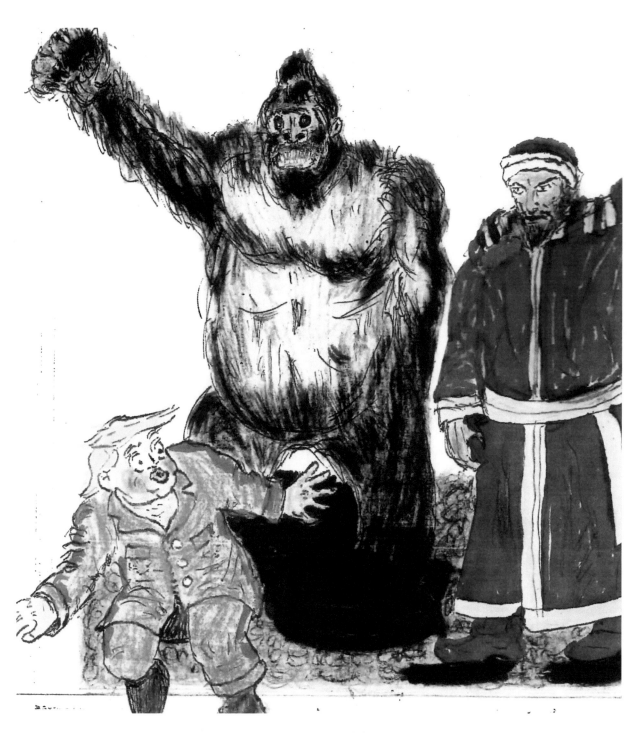

WHEN HE OPENS THE DOOR,
HE SUDDENLY FALLS TO THE FLOOR!

There stands a seven foot gorilla
And a sinister-looking Asian man in a hooded coat.
Von Grumpstein tries to get up
But his legs seem to float.
The gorilla helps him to a
Chair, as part of the plan.
The Asian man says, "My name is
One Odd Pan."

"My name is Furnigore" says,
The huge ape-like speaker.
We came because we heard you
Murdered my old high school teacher."

Von Grumpstein is stunned
Beyond belief.
He knew he was having a dream and would
Soon wake up, what a relief.

Pan says, "You have angered my friend
And you have plenty to fear.
Why did you kill one
He holds so dear?"

Furnigore looks angerly at
Von Grumpstein and says,
"You better start talking
Or you'll be dead."

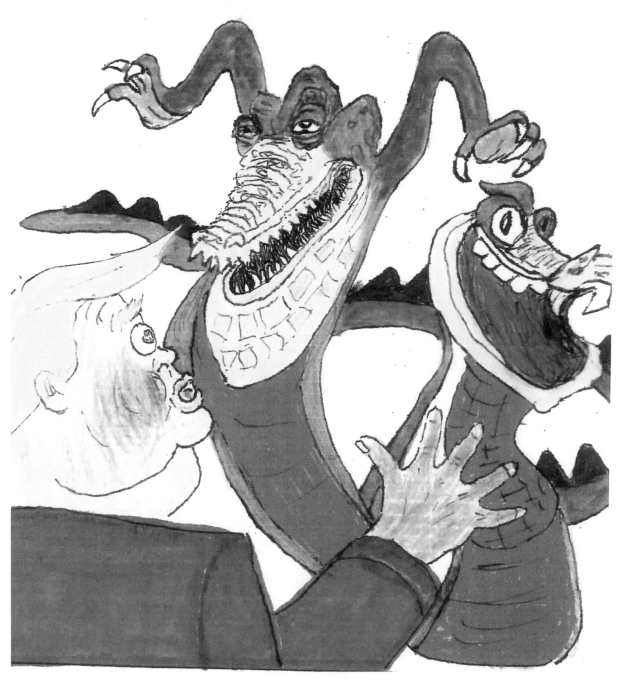

PAN SAYS, "WE HAVE SOME FRIENDS OUTSIDE
WE WOULD LIKE YOU TO MEET."

"It was a terrible accident.
We had no intention of killing her.
She fell and was severely hurt.
Her ailing heart would not stir."

"So, you admit you planned
To injure her." says Pan.
"I admit nothing, you have nothing on me.
No jury will believe you and your friend.
I will go free."

Pan says, "We have some friends outside
We would like you to meet.
Prepare yourself. Hold onto your seat.
Their names are Corky the Crocodile
And his brother Lisle."

"Do you really think a jury would believe
A gorilla that talks, and two
Lizards that talk and walk?"
The two lizards entered the room
And lunged at Von Grumpstein.
He leaped out of his chair
And started to scream.

His wife came into the room and said,
"Arnold, you're dreaming, get back into bed."
He said, "Wait till you hear the
Dream I just had!"

ARNOLD VON GRUMPSTEIN TOLD HIS BOARD OF DIRECTORS,
"I'LL DENY, AND DENY, AND DENY. I'LL JUST LIE AND LIE."

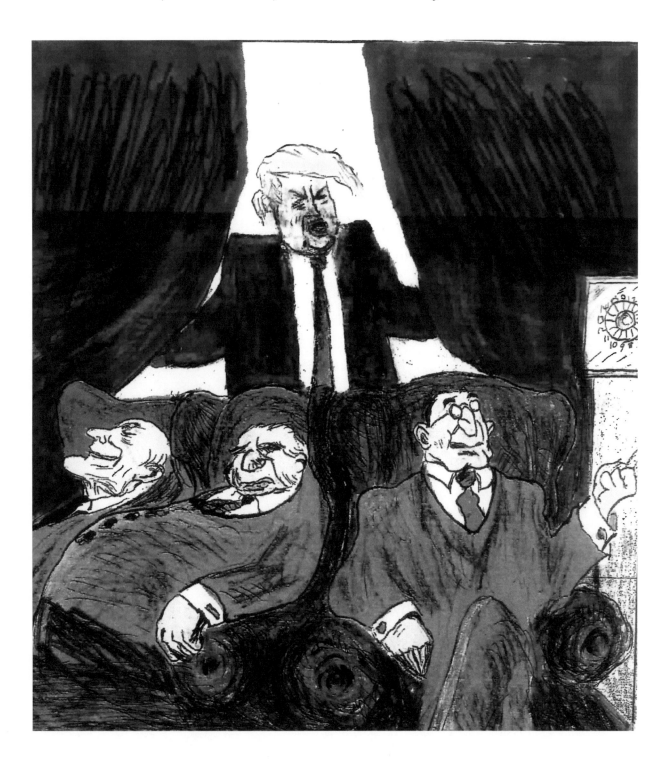

The next day, Von Grumpstein
Was visited by the F.B.I.
He was told they found out about his
Plan, and about his lie.

He was being held for murder
In the first degree.
He says, "I'm not worried;
I will go free!"

Arnold Von Grumpstein told his Board of Directors,
"I will deny, deny, and deny…
They have very little circumstantial evidence,
I'll just lie and lie and lie."

The trial begins and the prosecutors
And defense present their cases.
Even though the State had good evidence,
It lacked a firm basis.

In our system, evidence must be proved beyond
A reasonable doubt.
When defenders lie and deny, it confuses the
Jury, and it forgets what the trial is all about.

Just when it appeared that
Von Grumpsteen would go free,
The prosecutor says, "I have more
Witnesses I want you to see."

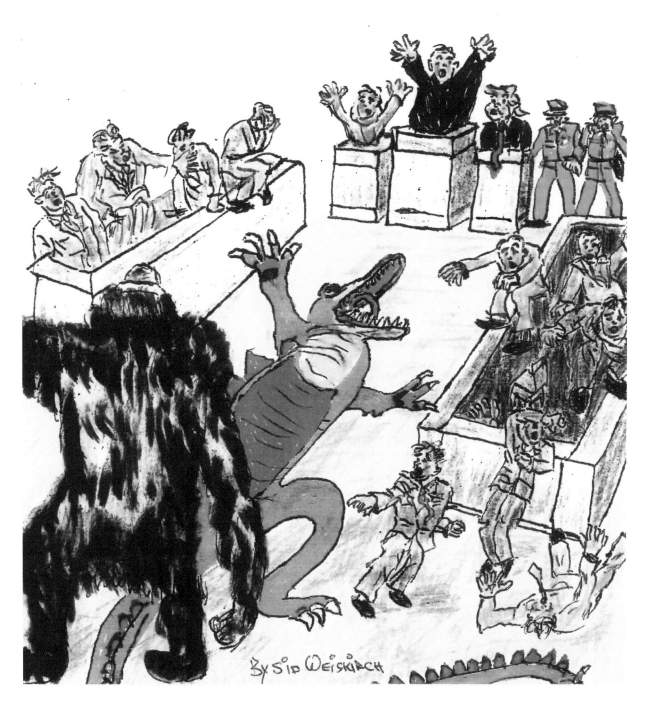

THE JUDGE SCREAMED,
"MISTRIAL"—"MISTRIAL"—"MISTRIAL"

There was a big commotion in the back of the room.
Furnigore, dressed as a gorilla, Corky, and Lisle,
raced up to the jury and the judge,
Screaming like a South Pacific typhoon.

Von Grumpstein froze, and could not believe his eyes.
The judge and all the jury ran for their lives.
There was nothing but screams and cries.

The judge declared a mistrial
And Von Grumpstein was free.
Furnigore, Corky, and Lisle
Disappeared after their spree.

Larry and his father sit down and feel badly
About what they have just seen.
They say they should have never allowed Pan
To propose such a crazy scheme.

When suddenly, Von Grumpstein comes
Up to them and said,
"I'll never forget what I've just seen. I'm sorry
For what I did and the life I have led.

I'm going to give $30 million to the Alzheimer's
Foundation to fund a research campaign
To prove biofeedback can help Alzheimer's
Patients relieve their pain.

"I will also give another 100-million-dollars
To build a hospital that will treat Alzheimer's
Patients FREE whenever they are ready.

"And use the Biofeedback treatments you
Started with your wife Letty."

THE END

EPILOGUE

A NEW 40-YEAR SWEDISH RESEARCH STUDY FOUND THAT WOMEN WHO EXERCISED REGULARLY HAD A 90 PERCENT LESS CHANCE OF GETTING ALZHEIMER'S IN THEIR SENIOR YEARS.

A large nursing home in Illinois is starting to use a biofeedback program to help their residents.

The National Football League is using a biofeedback program to help football players with concussion-related dementia. (see Denver Broncos)

All these things would not have happened without the sacrifices of Letty and other Alzheimer's patients, plus the help of One Odd Pan and Furnigore, from a country called the Clean Up Kingdom, in an alternate universe near our own. (This according to our own scientists and… The String Theory.)

In detail, this is my daily routine. I have done this for about 60 years every day. My wife (who was an executive social worker at the time) read it in a book by a doctor.

I do it for about a minute, three times a day. If I forget and something stressful happens, I could start seeing the flashing lights for about 15 minutes before the actual headache and ill feelings started. If I stopped and started the one minute exercise, the headache and lights went away. It really works.

First, I concentrate on my fingertips in both hands for a few seconds. I then start saying the trigger word (any word is okay). Mine is "vasodilate." After saying or thinking it for about 15 seconds, I begin to feel a tingling in my fingertips. I start counting up to 60 or 70. About half way through, I begin to feel my pulse beating in my fingertips.

That's it. Three times a day. It takes about two weeks of practice to get to the point when your pulse beat is very clear in both hands.

The doctor in the book explains the way it works as follows: He says everyone has a fight or flight process in our bodies the same as the animals in the jungle. When a serious danger comes up, the body rushes blood to the arms and legs to fight or run. After the danger is over, the blood rushes back to the brain and other places. This causes a migraine in SOME PEOPLE, like me. The biofeedback exercise mimics the blood rushing to the brain, only MILDER. This, he says, sort of dissolves the big rush of blood and sort of smooths it out. Thus, avoiding the headache.

My theory is this: If a person can cause the blood to rush to the brain three times a day, every day, I think it might clear the plaque and fog that develops in older people who do not have dangerous or stressful situations that younger people have every day.

WHAT WENT BEFORE AND WHAT COMES LATER

Book One - Furnigore & Larry

Furnigore and Larry is about an 8-year-old boy who liked to watch scary television shows. He falls asleep in a department store while his parents and his sister Val are buying a bed for his room. He dreams he is awakened by an ape-like, furniture-eating creature in the store. The creature's name is Furnigore, and he talks. Larry is very frightened and keeps Furnigore amused with jokes and riddles. Finally, he incurs Furnigore's anger with one of his jokes. Just as Furnigore is about to catch him, Larry is awakened by his mother. Larry tells everyone the fantastic story about Furnigore and how real it all seemed. He swears he will never watch another scary TV show as long as he lives.

Book Two - More Adventures of Furnigore.

Val, Larry's little sister, wants very badly to meet Furnigore, but she is told over and over that it was all a dream. Years later, when she is nine, she and a friend named Carly are playing with a chemistry set. There is an explosion, and the girls are knocked unconscious. They are transported to a strange world where they are found by One Odd Pan, an Asian-like sorcerer, who is President of a country called the Clean Up Kingdom. This prosperous land is blessed by nature with animals that keep the country clean and spic and span. These animals also talk. There is Wembly, the Woodpecker, whose birds eat old boats; Candice the

Cow, whose cows eat old computers; Humphry, the Horse, whose team eats old houses; and, of course, the head of the Clean Up Crew, Furnigore, who eats old furniture. The girls are kidnapped by a group called the Dust Catcher Mob. They are part of an evil group that accumulates junk and sells it to a country called Terrordom. Terrordom turns the junk into weapons and sells them to warring nations. The girls escape in a small boat and are being hunted when One Odd Pan conjures up a storm to cover a raid by Furnigore and his group of patrol boats out to rescue the girls. Huge waves overturn the girl's boat just as they wake up in a hospital. Val tells the family of the adventures with Pan and Furnigore. When she is told it is all another dream, she cannot believe it. Then, her friend Carly, who was with her throughout the adventure, also wakes up in the hospital's next room. Carly tells every one of her strange dream. It is exactly the same as Val's dream…This still remains an unexplained mystery to this day.

Book Three - Furnigore-Chase-Nate & Jake

Many years pass, and Val has a son named Chase. Chase and his two cousins, Nate and Jake, are dozing in their grandfather's backyard after a strenuous tennis lesson from grandfather. Suddenly, there appears an Asian gentleman named One Odd Pan who asks for their help in planning a large music and food festival in his far-off land called the Clean Up Kingdom. The teenage boys agree because of their experience with large Chicago and Milwaukee fests of this kind. Knowledge from their family's experience in sales, music, and organizational planning is why they were singled out by One Odd Pan.

After organizing and training the Clean Up Kingdom crew, the events go off perfectly until the end. A helicopter from Terrordom, the hated enemy of the Clean Up Kingdom, appears and spews smoke and coal dust all over the festival park. Furnigore gets Wembly the Woodpecker's crew to punch holes into the helicopter, and it crashes. After a huge explosion, the boys are awakened by Chase's mother. She says the sprinklers somehow got turned on and showered the boys. But, no one could explain how the boys had gotten covered with coal dust all over their bodies. The boys all had the same story about One Odd Pan, Furnigore, and the Clean Up Festival.

Val, Chase's mother, sees an image of One Odd Pan in a passing cloud and says, "Oh, no, not that dream again. Once in a lifetime should be enough."

Book Four - Furnigore and Karen

One Odd Pan has a problem with his restaurant chain. It's losing money. He and his cousins need outside help to get the restaurants back into the black. He finally chooses Karen Hall, head chef at a Boca Raton Florida hotel. He appears to her in a dream and makes her an offer she cannot refuse.

She comes to the Clean Up Kingdom and immediately makes the needed corrections—to the poorly managed chain. Just as she is about to leave, a new chain opens up that threatens the health and welfare of the Kingdom. She discovers a connection to Terrordom, the arch enemy of One Odd Pan. Furnigore and his team plant a sound recording device with the help of Wembly, the Woodpecker. They discover a secret plot to poison the people of the Clean Up Kingdom. With this information, they are able to thwart the plot and close down the rival restaurants. One Odd Pan says he will grant Karen three wishes. But she awakens back in Florida and is about to forget the whole weird dream when a messenger delivers a strange large box. When she gets it open, she finds it is full of money for her own restaurant and her other two wishes. A note explains the money is from an unclaimed Swiss bank account, so she is in the clear. The note is signed by none other than O.O.P...One Odd Pan!

Book Five - Furnigore Solves the Y2K Problem

Again One Odd Pan must seek the help of the boys when all computers crash in the Cleanup Kingdom after January 1, 2000. There is no heat or power. All activity comes to a stop. The people go back to the days of the wild, wild west. No one had prepared for this problem. Meanwhile, wealthy computer manufacturers have stolen a disc which could solve the computer problem. They are holding it until Pan agrees to replace all present computers with new ones from the computer manufacturers. Furnigore and the boys try a variety of ways to solve the problem, but have no luck, until Furnigore uses the chicken soup system on the computers. By combining all the methods with special power from a casino gambling ship, they finally resolve the problem after heroics from Furnigore to steal the disc back from the manufacturers.

Book Six - Furnigore Runs for President

One Odd Pan's term as president is expiring. Furnigore is running for president against an opponent who will take away many of the benefits enjoyed by a majority of the average citizens of the Cleanup Kingdom. He will work for the wealthy and for the dishonest members of the Kingdom. Furnigore and One Odd Pan seek help from Larry and his friends and relatives because they have helped in the past.

A famous political consultant is recruited to help Furnigore get elected. After many twists and turns, Robert Hole, Furnigore's opponent, has his past personal errors exposed on national TV. Furnigore wins the election and his consultant gets a surprise bonus. His wife, who is his arch rival in Washington, suddenly becomes his partner after she is relieved of her job with the opposing party. (One Odd Pan and Clarice the computer wizard did a little political chicanery to make this happen.)

Book Seven - Furnigore and the C201 Cure

This time, Larry, who now teaches biology, and the cousins, who are all in premed courses, try to find a way to reach Furnigore and One Odd Pan. They remember that there is no disease called C201 in the Cleanup Kingdom. Since C201 has defied a cure here on Earth, they thought perhaps there might be a clue to the cure in the Kingdom. They luckily find a way to reach Furnigore, and after pursuing many research projects, they finally make a breakthrough. A clue comes from the DNA of senior citizens in the Kingdom, and the boys hurry back to Earth, with Pan's help, of course, to spread the word of their discovery.

CHASE THE BASS AND VLADIMERE RONGNOTESKI

Vladimer Rongnoteski is the conductor of the famous Boston Symphony Orchestra. Some of the members of this great classical orchestra want to play more modern and popular music to attract a younger audience. He has many arguments with the members, and after one of the more arduous ones, he retires for a rest. He dozes off and has a dream where a large bass violin and other instruments come to life and demand he play more contemporary music. He is adamant, and he believes these instruments mean to harm him. He runs away, and he is chased to the highest ramparts of Orchestra Hall. He leaps onto a huge chandelier to escape the charging instruments. As he is about to fall into the crowd, he awakens from the feverish dream.

He is so moved by the experience that he decides to form a new orchestra. And so, the Boston Pops Orchestra was born, at least that was one story of how it happened.

Book Eight - Furnigore and Vladimere Rongnoteski

Furnigore and One Odd Pan ask Larry and his cousins for advice once again at a family reunion. They are in a program to bring a symphony orchestra to their Clean Up Kingdom. They have local and country type musicians, but no classical training.

Larry and the group recommend they contact Vladimere Rongnoteski, the conductor of world famous orchestras, to take control of Furnigore's project. After appearing before a frightened Rongnoteski in a dream, they offer him a reward of three wishes if he can give the Kingdom a symphony orchestra within a year. Knowing he is dreaming, Rongnoteski agrees to go. He asks for enough money for a new symphony hall, a new summer pavilion, and a new training Civic Orchestra.

After many months of disappointments and frustration, the first concert was about to begin. Pan realizes it would be a terrible failure, so he uses the last of his tragic potion to make the musicians play brilliantly. Rongnoteski brings in a new team of teachers and is successful in completing the rest of the season.

Everyone was pleased, and Rongnoteski awoke back in his home city and went back to his regular rehearsals and concerts. He knew he had a very unusual dream and simply forgot all about it. Months later, he finds a note under his door with only a series of numbers written on it. On a whim, he purchases a $1.00 lottery ticket for the huge five state lottery using the numbers on the ticket. He faints when he realizes he has the winning ticket and the money to complete his three wishes in the dream.

Larry hears about Rongnoteski winning the lottery and has kept up with the concerts in the Cleanup-Kingdom, He asks Rongnoteski to admit the existence of Furnigore and One Odd Pan so that everyone will know his adventures in the Cleanup Kingdom actually happened. Rongnoteski tells him it is impossible because the money will have to be returned, and the world will lose the new symphony hall, the new summer pavilion, and the great new training ground for new musicians at the new Civic Orchestra. Larry agrees, and Pan and Furnigore's existence still remains a secret to all, except Larry, his relatives and, of, course, Vladimere Rongnoteski.

Book Nine - Furnigore and Hannah

Larry and his wife, Debbie, have a 20-month-old daughter named Hannah. Her grandfather thinks she is extremely bright. (As all grandparents do.) But, after a dream, he believes Hannah has extraordinary powers coming from their old friend One Odd Pan. In the dream, Hannah says she will deny everything. She tells grandfather that Pan wants to keep tabs on Larry and his cousins because they have been so helpful to his kingdom in the past. She says Pan gave her powers of intelligence and speech, so she can report to him.

On September 11, 2001, America is attacked and goes to war. Larry's cousins are all in the reserves and are sent to the war zone. Grandfather makes sure to discuss the war with Larry in the presence of Hannah. Soon, Larry himself has a dream about Pan and Furnigore. They tell Larry they will help with the war by giving Larry information about troop movements. He must tell America's president that he can provide vital information for winning the war. Larry goes to Washington, and after overcoming many obstacles, he finally convinces the president to use the secret information. Using the information from Larry, America wins the war quickly. The president tells Larry he will keep the source of the information secret if he can contact him later if it becomes necessary. The next day the president receives a message on his most secret Telefax machine. It says, "Remember it was all a dream." Signed Furnigore and One Odd Pan.

Book Ten - Furnigore and the String Theory

All of Larry's children are grown and in colleges following their advanced studies with their cousins.

They are all gathered at their grandfather's house. They talk about their adventures in the Cleanup Kingdom with Furnigore and One Odd Pan.

They talk about how the human race evolved and other deep subjects when the question of how they came to be involved with Furnigore kept mystifying them. They decided to ask Larry to get Dr. Droid to transfer them out to the Cleanup Kingdom again.

Dr. Droid only agrees if they finally tell him where they go and who the devil were Furnigore and One Odd Pan and all his relatives. After they arrive, Pan tells them he uses his magic potion to send them back to Earth, but he has no idea how Dr. Droid is able to send them to the Cleanup Kingdom. Pan's potion is in very short supply, and it only came to him by accident. He doesn't know how to replenish it.

Pan explains the String Theory. He says there are tiny particles in the universe that collide. When they do, they form parallel worlds. We cannot feel or hear them, but they exist. Pan's formula allows him to pass through the worlds. Dr. Droid's equipment can send Larry's relatives out, but not back to our universe.

Everyone is shocked to realize their adventures were actually true and not dreams contacted by hypnosis or computers.

Later, when they are all back in Dr. Droid's lab, Larry can't convince Dr. Droid of the facts he presents to him. So, they go on into the night trying to explain the unexplainable.

Book Eleven - Furnigore and Ben

This book is a about Larry's son, Ben, now an astronaut commanding the first manned trip to Mars.

The trip is boring, and there are some jokes to amuse the crew during the long days of travel. Finally, they land and start their experiments on the long dead planet. Suddenly, their ship is bombarded with electric rays and storms so bad, that it looks like the rocket will be destroyed.

Larry calls on Dr. Droid to contact Ben on Mars. One Odd Pan and Furnigore have determined that Ben's ship has been attacked by Martians, who live in underground cities hidden from view and from the poisonous planet above. They give Ben a radio channel to speak to the commander, General Jesicus.

The surprised general tells Ben that Martians have observed the earth for hundreds of years. They have seen how Europeans and Americans have treated and enslaved Africans, South Americans, and American Indians.

They want no part of any further rocket expeditions. Ben makes a deal with the general, and he is allowed to leave...and never come back. Thus ending the exploration of the Martian planet.

Book Twelve - Furnigore and Curley

Grandfather and his 11-year-old neighbor Curley go to the local zoo. While there, they visit the new gorilla exhibit which has a large family of apes and gorillas living there just like they do in the forests of Africa. The visitors circle far above in a long circular viewing area. The crowds are huge and excited. Curley accidentally falls into the gorilla's living area. This causes panic above and in the gorilla section. Large gorillas think Curley is a danger to the children and threaten him. A mother gorilla protects Curley as much as she can. Grandfather is in a panic too. He calls for help from his connections to Furnigore and One Odd Pan. Pan sends Furnigore to the gorilla compound to help Curley. He has to confront the main gorilla, and after much negotiating, they decide to have a hand to hand combat to decide what will happen to Curley. Furnigore wins and disappears while Grandfather and Curley leave for home. The major in charge of the rescue team can't understand what happened. Grandfather tells him to ask the President of the United States. He will explain it all to him,

Book Thirteen - Furnigore and the Escaped Convicts

Two convicts escape from the State Prison and are on the run for thirty days. The search turns up nothing...Meanwhile, Grandfather and his neighbor Curly are in a nationwide bird counting contest.

They go into the neighboring deep woods because of the abundance of rare birds among the tallest trees in their area. The person spotting the most birds will win a large prize, so they spend a great deal of time searching the trees. Curly gets excited spotting a rare owl and runs off, away from Grandfather. Grandfather can't keep up, and Curly has disappeared among the trees. After several hours, Grandfather calls his son Larry for help when he discovers Curly tied to a tree with the two convicts in their camp.

The situation becomes desperate when it starts raining, and Grandfather's cell phone battery starts to run down. Larry calls One Odd Pan and Furnigore for help. Using all his magic, Pan sends Wembly the Woodpecker and friends to harass the convicts. Later, he sends Furnigore to finish the job, which he does in true Furnigore style. The battered convicts are turned over to the police and the headlines the next day say…

SENIOR CITIZEN AND 11-YEAR-OLD BOY SUBDUE AND DISARM KILLERS…What a way to end a huge man hunt this way. How they did it remains a mystery until this day.

Any earnings the author will receive from the sales of this book will go into a fund to train caregivers and biofeedback practitioners to work with Alzheimer's patients FREE OF CHARGE. Hopefully, many others will start using the daily exercises as a preventative from getting dementia and Alsheimer's in their future senior years.

Questions will be answered by email at: weiskirch@att.net

CPSIA information can be obtained
at www.ICGtesting.com
Printed in the USA
BVHW022240140121
597886BV00011B/23